COLLISION WITH SELF, A REMEDY

A GUIDE TO MENTAL WELLNESS

JANICE E. DALER

authorHOUSE®

AuthorHouse™
1663 Liberty Drive
Bloomington, IN 47403
www.authorhouse.com
Phone: 1-800-839-8640

This book and the process shared within are not intended as medical, psychiatric, or
otherwise professional advice. This is intended only as an actual experience to share
for the benefit of others. It is regarding the confusion and negative emotions that can
sometimes overwhelm a person dealing with the typical but many demands of life, and
how to overcome them. This book is not intended for any matters above and beyond
that. If you have been mistreated or abused physically, mentally, emotionally, or
otherwise, seek professional advice to guide you through the effects of that burden.

Published by AuthorHouse   12/23/2014

ISBN: 978-1-4969-5516-6 (sc)
ISBN: 978-1-4969-5515-9 (e)

Library of Congress Control Number: 2014921198

Any people depicted in stock imagery provided by Thinkstock are models,
and such images are being used for illustrative purposes only.
Certain stock imagery © Thinkstock.

This book is printed on acid-free paper.

Because of the dynamic nature of the Internet, any web addresses or links contained in
this book may have changed since publication and may no longer be valid. The views
expressed in this work are solely those of the author and do not necessarily reflect the
views of the publisher, and the publisher hereby disclaims any responsibility for them.

CONTENTS

To all of humanity.

We're doing the best that we can
with what we've got to work with,
or through, as the case sometimes may be.

PROLOGUE

Dear Reader, if you have decided to buy this book or someone close to you has purchased it for you, then let me begin by saying *hang in there*. Because it can only mean that you are in a difficult place. The very good news is that you are self-aware enough (or someone else takes enough of a loving interest in you) to notice that you're not yourself and can use a little help. I can empathize and sympathize, as I have been there. But I've also made it up from that low point, and I want to tell you: this new place in life is not only so much better than where I've just come from, but I'm even tempted to say I'm the best I've ever been.

I won't belabor the point for you here because I remember the state of mind you're currently in, and that it feels like you don't have a lot of time to spare. I will share my journey in the pages to follow in minimal fashion, so that you know I really can empathize with you. Then I'm sharing in greater detail the remedies and practices that helped me get me out of that low point, particularly as it relates to a Meditation on Words.

Please understand that these practices are what worked for me. From them please use what works for you, and don't try so hard with those things that don't feel like a fit. By all means personalize the practices to meet your individual situation and needs. But most of all, stick with it.

I now know from experience that we can help our own mind change with repeated exercise, not unlike the way we can change the muscles of our bodies by going regularly to the gym. Similarly, both take time so, again, please stick with it to get the results.

You'll be happy that you did, and that happiness is the ultimate point to all of this.

INTRODUCTION

"Be careful, sweetheart," she warned me time and time again. "The universe is trying to get your attention."

Now that I have gone through and emerged from *exactly* what she was warning me about, I can tell you this: she was right; my attention was definitely caught.

I can also tell you with great certainty that if you are lucky enough, as I was, to have a friend who cares enough to pay that kind of attention to you; enough to give you fair warning—heed it! And consider that friend a *major* blessing in your life. She or he may even be the one who gave you this book as an expression of concern for your well-being.

As for my friend, her name is Michele. She is French, in her seventies as of the writing of this page, and experienced beyond her years. She not only lives life, she is a student of it: constantly observing how it unfolds, taking mental notes, and applying the lessons day by day. She is willing to share these lessons if you've got the time to lend her your ear, as I love to do. And it was she who warned me many times of what was to come, while she bore witness to my life and actions as only a true friend can do.

I was unable to heed her warnings of my pending downward spiral, because I could not understand it until I experienced it. It's an unfortunate way that we sometimes need to learn. She later came to call my experience a "collision with my self."

As for myself, my name is Janice, and this is not so much the story about how I collided with my self, but more about the things I did to emerge from the crash. My story is not dramatic or traumatic but pretty run-of-the-mill stuff ... which is precisely why I thought I should share it.

It seems to me this kind of collision with self is happening, or poised to happen, to people all around me. It strikes me as an end result of the way of the world these days: we are a generally overworked, overstressed, multitasking, unbalanced, unhealthy society. That combination of overages has consequences. Or, as Michele put it: the universe (or your world as you know it) will eventually get your attention to let you know something's got to give. If you don't take the action to adjust, the action will be taken for you—and you will crash. That is how the issue was forced for me.

When you get to that crashing point, it's a low one: dark, messy, confusing, and despairing. It takes time and effort to unravel the mess that, by my experience, can take months or years to create. This book is therefore intended as a map, in a sense, to help show you the way up from the bottom.

Not all of the methods and processes shared here may work for you, but they should collectively help get you going in the right direction. As you notice benefits from one method or the other you can capitalize upon it in ways that do work for you. It is my hope that the Meditation on Words has a noticeable positive impact for you. It is that "workout for the brain" that I personally learned to be the most imperative part of my climb out of the crash and of my continued success going forward. It's what made me most conscious of my relationship to my brain, and I now tend to this relationship on a daily basis.

Importantly, I wanted to put this information out there to help other people heed the warning they might need to hear, or to not give up hope if they've already collided with self, or to take steps to get up from the low point and back to their "old self," only better. The most rewarding outcome is to emerge from the mental rubble with a clearer sense of self, and the direction you are headed with your life. Because I think the most valuable lesson I've learned from all of this is quite simple, but the essential key: *This is no one else's life but your own, and happiness is your choice.*

CHAPTER ONE

The Collision

My collision was years in the making before the ultimate crash. Like I mentioned before, it was nothing traumatic, just a mix of the usual stuff that is so prevalent in the world today: climbing the ladder at work, staying too late at the office, taking classes on top of working long hours, running the household, paying the bills, tending to family and friends, planning a wedding, losing time to take care of myself, losing track of just how unhealthy I had become, hitting middle age, and so on and so on. It was pile upon pile of too many things to do, and too little time to do them each and every day.

Add on top of the "usual stuff" some of the unique things personal to the timing of my situation and you've got a real collision course formula for disaster: I was an investment manager during the financial crash of 2008 and recently read a white paper regarding advisors suffering post-traumatic stress disorder as a result of that prolonged experience. My (now) husband and I had just purchased a new home at the peak of the real estate market and simultaneously could not sell the old one because of the subsequent crash in the housing market. My father was enduring multiple back-to-back surgeries. Then there was the news – the *constant* stream of negative headline news forthcoming every single day: Bear Sterns, the Lehman event, the market crash, the threat of a run on the banks, the announcement of economic stimulus, the imminent end of one US presidential term, the muckraking of election season, the election itself, unemployment figures, multiple wars, the economy, more stimulus, the Euro zone crisis, a US presidential term re-election, tsunamis, earthquakes, shootings, hurricanes, *more* shootings, the Mayan end of the world, the economy, the economy, the economy! The sheer amount of information, and the constant and various sources of it, was (and remains) utterly insane.

In addition to this global news was the constant flow of personal stories of distress: friends and family losing jobs, losing homes, losing life savings, losing husbands to deployment, losing health, everyone generally losing faith. If I wanted some good news I was going to have to turn over rocks and search for it, because none was coming my way during this time.

I started feeling affected by the constant flow of negative news and my all-consuming hours at the office in many insidious ways. It began with poor eating and exercise habits, which opened the door for more bad habits like too much drinking. My body started misbehaving in steady and compounding ways: stomach issues, jaws sore from teeth clenching, hair loss, and sleepless nights full of worry. I was consumed by anxiety in the form of a tight chest, getting out of bed at night to leave myself voice messages at the office, bouts of sudden and uncontrollable crying. I started to experience multiple injuries to an already-weakened body: a torn calf muscle, a "locked" muscle in my shoulder, a burning pain in the muscles of my forearm—on and on it went, including other physical issues too sensitive to mention here. The final piece, moderate depression, was different from the physical ailments, and something that I didn't recognize until it had been underway for a couple of months.

This realization came about by experiencing "flashes" of happiness from earlier times in my life, and noticing the stark contrast to my present state of mind. On the heels of that personal realization came four different people who felt the need to touch base with me and say, "You don't seem yourself," and to ask if everything was alright. Almost simultaneous with that experience was an emotional confrontation with my boss that was highly uncharacteristic of me.

It was the culmination of all of these "signals" that made me turn to my husband one Friday night and make the statement that signified my crash had come. We were walking down the main street of town together at the end of a grueling work week. As we passed the movie theatre marquee I had one of my flashbacks of a happier time in our life and relationship. The memory consisted of a summertime scene when we'd first met, and we were walking past that same marquee holding hands, laughing, and looking decidedly more happy and free than in the present moment. It was that flash of "how things once had been" interrupting my dire case of "how things are now" that caused me to suddenly stop, turn to my husband and say:

"I don't think I'm okay."

CHAPTER TWO

Baby Steps

The first thing I did following that personal statement of recognition was call my doctor to secure her next available appointment. She was amazing that day, while I was quite simply a mess. The uncontrollable tears were commonplace for me now and were on display in her office. I was falling apart in front of her, both figuratively and literally. Some descriptors I remember using with her to describe the current state of my life—or rather, my relationship to my life—included feeling as if I were "floating off into the distance like a helium balloon." I remember that image coming to me often during this depressed time, and I believe it was the visual representation of me not being in control of the direction of my life. Instead, the days and weeks were coming and going in haphazard fashion and I felt helpless to do anything other than watch myself float in whatever direction each daily set of demands would take me.

Another distinct perception was feeling on the outside looking in on my day-to-day actions. I was no longer connected to what I was doing; instead I was just going through the motions. I believe this was a direct reaction to how intense the demands had become on my emotional self so that a passive, stand-by attitude was all I could muster. I learned during this time how good an actress I can be for those around me (particularly colleagues and clients). I could outwardly say and do the right things on cue, even though internally I was standing on the precipice. I remember describing that lack of connectedness, for my doctor, as "a crack right down the center of my being." It was like I had been split open so that the soul of me (the joy of living) had somewhere along the way slipped out and disappeared.

She had known me for seventeen years and could easily tell that this "wasn't me," and that I was in a state of duress. She offered some sound advice that day that I will share here in two short but important statements:

- Number one: depression should be treated in a multi-faceted way as there can be many things contributing to it such as vitamin deficiencies, medications you are taking, hormonal imbalances, external forces, and more.
- Number two: important decisions are not to be made at your low and confused point (e.g., leaving your job, leaving your marriage). *They are best made from a position of strength and clarity.*

These were the two most meaningful pieces of advice I could have asked for, and they set the groundwork for me and my course for the many months to come. I left her office that day with a short-term and mid-term plan for getting myself back to a position of health, strength, and clarity from a physical standpoint, including a blood work series and follow-up, super doses of particular vitamins, a serotonin neurotransmitter booster, and more.

My doctor's recommendations also included ways to address the mental aspect of my need for strength and clarity. These included a leave of absence from work, counseling sessions, and a visit to see my family. My response to these recommendations was that I would call on her for that leave of absence letter, but that I was not prepared to leave her office with it in hand. I believe I needed it "dangling" out there as an absolute last resort in case I couldn't get clear and strong with the plan we just put into place. I wanted to give the physical measures a chance to work.

However, I did take her advice and immediately booked a trip home to see my family. They are my foundation and my counsel in life, and I enjoy and am comforted by my family relationships. I have always felt solidly "grounded" around them, something I was *desperately* in need of at this point.

As for professional counseling, I had done that before at various points in my life and know it to be an incredible help. I have often said to friends considering counseling that it's something everyone should do when they attain the age of thirty. It can help to sort through that first set of "growing-up years" and collecting experience, so that one can recognize what is *not* working (and get rid of it), and can understand what *is* working (and capitalize upon it). So, I certainly didn't set that recommendation aside that day because I don't believe in it. Rather, I vaguely knew that I had started to connect to that counseling need in myself and was working on it in my own way.

CHAPTER THREE

A Meditation on Words

Somewhere along the way to my crashing point I randomly pulled out and dusted off a sketch pad and drawing pencils from my college days. I hadn't touched these items in years. But when I stumbled upon them I decided to keep them downstairs by the television where my husband and I were spending too much time at night, after coming home from work and feeling "fried." At this point in the crash I needed the mindless escape of the TV to dull my troubled mind. But the commercials had become incessant and annoying, so I wanted something to do to avoid them altogether. During each commercial, I would pick up the sketch book and draw.

At first it started with simply putting colors and shapes on the page, not unlike creating a mandala[1] which is a focused mini-meditation in itself. I could immediately tell that this new habit was beneficial for my depressed mind.

This practice was giving me a concentrated focus on something other than the worries I had accumulated and was obsessing about – not in the brainless escape of TV, but instead with a specific intent. The intent was simple but positive: choosing colors and shapes that were pleasing to me.

---

[1] *Mandala: the word is from the classical Indian language of Sanskrit. Loosely translated to mean "circle," a mandala is far more than a simple shape ... and can be seen as a model for the organizational structure of life itself. (Excerpt from mandalaproject.org). In various spiritual traditions, mandalas are employed for focusing attention of aspirants and adepts, as a spiritual teaching tool, for establishing a sacred space, and as an aid to meditation and trance induction. (Excerpt from wikipedia.org).*

After a time I started adding words to the colors and shapes on the page: simple, positive words that I would have to *intently* concentrate on during the course of coloring them onto the page. I could tell this additional level of focus was even better for my troubled, negative mind.

As I engaged in this habit I became increasingly aware that it was helping me to get out of my head by intercepting my constant stream of depression. Like the flashes of happiness mentioned earlier, drawing also made me aware of how my mind had been carrying on before I interrupted it. My highly negative, depressed thoughts were the main source of perspective and energy coursing through me, and they *clearly* needed to change. My mindset was affecting *everything*. I soon moved from awareness to true understanding that I needed to continue and expand upon this exercise for my brain. The drawings and words were going to be the way I'd now send messages to myself to change my state of mind … to slowly and habitually turn it around from the incessantly negative back to the positive. I dubbed this new practice a "Meditation on Words."

As the impact of this Meditation on Words became clearer to me, my next level of comprehension was that the pages needed to come out of the sketch pad and onto some surface where I would read them every day, multiple times per day. By doing this I would accomplish two things: 1) repeatedly arrest the current, negative thoughts and habits of my brain and 2) immediately replace that arrested space with new, positive thoughts for my brain.

In our home that location could only be one place: the refrigerator doors. In my upbringing they are the "command central" of households across the nation: peppered with save-the-date info, notes, schedules, shopping lists, and more. Many people now use their phone for these types of reminders, but in our home the fridge still has its place. It is the first destination I stumble to every morning for juice; the last stop every night for a drink before bed; and about fifty times in between … every single day. This was *precisely* the kind of repetition I was seeking and so it is where my sketch pad drawings started to live.

The interesting thing about command central in our home is that it had already been serving as what I'd call "communication central" for my husband and me. We had previously established the habit of leaving notes and phrases on the fridge to communicate with each other. This is because (for my husband in particular) notes take away the intimidating edge of confrontation in face-to-face discussions that all married couples need to have when working through the business of life. So now he, too, was regularly seeing my sketch pad images of positive thinking. These images eventually became more broadly focused on depicting the life imagined for the both of us. The effect was both interesting and powerful. I was too bogged down in my own woes to see that the negative energy I was bringing into our household was infectious, and having an impact on my husband's days as well. Likewise, the images of positive thinking I was posting onto command central were equally infectious. The positive reinforcement that I was seeing fifty times per day was also turning my husband's underlying mind toward the positive as well. Importantly, we were now being reminded of the same ideas for our life together at the same time. This brought us onto the same page with our day-to-day decision-making processes.

As an example, one of the determinations necessary to get myself back on track physically was to eat healthier. I had depleted my body of basic nutrients and minerals through years of very poor eating habits. Late nights and long hours at the office made it not at all uncommon for a bag of chips and a few beers to be our evening meal. That, coupled with some of our personal uncertainties about the food industry in general, led to the following Meditation on Words: "Real Food, Locally Grown." Within this newly stated agreement we were equally conscious to grab a bag of organic carrots and some hummus instead of chips and beer, after a late night at the office.

Another reinforcement came from a year-end Meditation on Words that we did together in 2012. In preparation for the New Year and what we intended to be a new era, we came up with a whole series of Meditations on Words to guide us, and hung it on the refrigerator. It's like a poster, full of more than a dozen phrases, one of which is "More Outdoors, Less Indoors." He and I originally moved to Colorado with intent, because we both love the outdoors. In my husband's case, I would go so far as to say he *needs* the outdoors to maintain his sanity. The unbalanced life we had worked ourselves into—with far too much time spent sitting in the controlled, false environment of our offices—was literally killing us. That statement is not to be taken lightly. We were indisputably becoming the poster children for a heart attack at middle age: weight gain, high stress, high cholesterol, prescribed to Lipitor, no exercise, too much drinking, unhealthy eating, bad sleeping habits, and so on.

With the daily presence of that new reminder "talking" to us from command central we were prompted to seek and accept every outdoor opportunity that came our way, even though we had grown ridiculously out of shape. Amazingly, the more opportunities we took the more that came our way. As an example, after years of not going on hut trips (which is skiing to a cabin in the woods for an overnight stay) we had two back-to-back, completely random offers in one month from people we hardly knew … and we took them both! This started to change our identities from "couch potatoes" back to active outdoor people, and our decisions and expectations of ourselves (and each other) followed suit.

One addition to our year-end meditation that was suggested by my husband was "More Romance." He was much more specific in how he originally phrased this, but I toned it down a little since command central would be seen by all who entered our home. I mention it here for the masses because the business of life can turn your marriage into feeling exactly like that: all business. The meaning of "romance" can span a wide spectrum of what you want that to be (more intimacy, more travel, more spontaneity, more one-on-one time, etc.). So a little reminder from one partner to another of how you can and should still have fun together is an important thing.

While maintaining the practice of posting each Meditation on Words to command central, I started to add other mental exercises to each day to increase the workout for my brain. I was growing keenly aware of and connected to my state of mind, and understood that this connection was the key to my quality of life. I was starting to learn that I could control my mind, instead of be controlled by it. However, while I recognized the immediate benefits of the Meditation on Words, I was still a very long way off from a healthy state of mind. My recovery to positive thinking was a multi-month process that had to work through many layers of personal examination. But I did eventually return myself to a positive state of being through the individual and compounding impact of all of these things in conjunction with the Meditation on Words: morning meditation, the practice of forgiveness, going back to church (for a short time), deep-breathing exercises, going often on a Thankful Walk[2], reading *The Daily Word* (a gift to me from Michele; it is a bi-monthly publication of daily affirmations), and more.

---

[2] *Thankful Walk is the practice of a 15 to 20-minute meditative walk in which you use the entire time to list in your mind, one by one, slowly and with great intent, the things you are thankful for in life. It can include all things big and small, from being thankful for the beautiful weather of that particular day, to being thankful for the health of your loved ones, and everything in between. The idea is to turn your mind to the positive in a repetitive, focused fashion.*

Though I have listed these commitments concisely, I should clarify that I took them on with unwavering dedication and great determination. The quality of my life absolutely depended on my devotion to these practices. It was around this time that I often reminded myself to never, never, never give up, no matter what life may bring. So these were not actions I tried to do with a random, here-and-there kind of frequency; I did these things habitually, every day and multiple times per day wherever appropriate. To illustrate: it was the pastor of my church who suggested during a morning sermon the practice of forgiveness. He explained that it needed to be done three times per day for twenty-one consecutive days. So I took on his challenge, because I realized the need to forgive was one that personally applied to me (I was blaming others for the state of mental distress I was in), and I did not miss a single session for all twenty-one consecutive days.

Eventually, about four months into my everyday commitments, I found myself one morning feeling so full of gratitude for how happy and positive I felt that I was actually *giving thanks* for having crashed to my low point. That low point of desperation is what gave me the opportunity to recognize my relationship to my brain so that I could understand and commit to the process of taking better care of it. Losing my positive state of mind—the filter for how I perceived and therefore lived my life—and having to fight so hard to get it back made me appreciate it more than ever before. I now understood how much my personal happiness was something I had been taking for granted. I did not know until this experience that it could be so deeply lost, or how much dedicated effort it would take to get it back. I was so surprised to hear myself give thanks for something that felt so desperate and dislocated at the beginning that I knew I was better now than I had ever been before: happier, peaceful, grounded, more experienced in understanding my mind, and better prepared for the next curve ball that Life would inevitably throw at me.

It was that last part—knowing that at some point I'd be challenged by my circumstances again—that led me to write this little book. It's not only a future reminder for me to recall what I've learned, but something to share with everyone else who may find themselves at the low point of their own collision with self. I've come to realize in this day and age that the collision is as universal as is catching the common cold. I already see it in the micro-universe of my friends and loved ones, so for the population at large I am considering the possibility of self-collision strong. Based on the continuous flow of shocking headline news about how people are acting out these days, I would say self-collisions are happening all around us on a more frequent basis. These headlines make me believe that our society is disconnected from the concept of taking care of our state of mind, and simultaneously losing the skill of coping mechanisms for the daily hurdles in life. Therefore, it wasn't a question of *why would I* write this book; it was more the inability to offer a good answer to the question of *why wouldn't I* share it with all?

CHAPTER FOUR

The Lesson

The next section of this book is a selection of phrases that were posted on our command central, provided here to help you start your own Meditation on Words: the workout for your brain. Grab some colored pencils and spend some time *sincerely* focusing on the words and phrases. Let your mind do more than just see the words and meanings; concentrate on their message and allow your thoughts to "marinate" in them for a while. Remember that I used this word-meditation time as a replacement for commercials … I didn't want to zone out on the TV during a long string of sixty-second spots, so I zoned *in* on my meditations and repeated them often throughout the evening—for easily twenty minutes each night on a consistent basis.

If you want to do as I did (see *Appendix*), spend time coloring the words, drawing imagery around the words, adding colors to emphasize the words; the whole point is to give your brain ample opportunity to connect to the meaning of the words. And then, after you've spent your time meditating on the words, post the pages to the command central of your home. Or take a picture of each Meditation on Words and create it as the wallpaper for your smart phone or other hand-held device (or do both). Given how often we look at our phones, this level of repetition will also suffice. The positive messages need to be where your brain will repetitively see them to arrest negative thoughts and be re-trained in how to think.

It may seem such a simple and small practice, and in actuality it is. But my experience tells me this: if your collision is anything like mine was, you're going to have to start with your foundation and work up from there in baby steps. The mind is a *powerful* piece of the puzzle that needs to be put back in its place after the crash, and you have to do so by giving it something positive to do, often.

The majority of these words are the basic ones that helped me through the very first phase of my process, in which it felt like there was a permanent crack in my rose-colored glasses: *everything was negative* for me. A razor-sharp focus on the positive was therefore my starting place and the number one goal. I recognize now that I had months, and to some extent years, of a negative mind habit to unwind, so that is why the words were simple and the meaning was so targeted.

The larger phrases included herein came about as I understood more of what I was trying to change in my mind's habits. As you see these phrases, such as "focus on your mind's self-talk," think about them. Everyone has an underlying self-talk going on in their mind, and it's a powerful current in your perception. Have you checked in with it lately to see what it's telling you on a constant basis? Is it a positive or negative feedback? Or perhaps it's a constant flow of worry or resentment? Whatever it may be, if it's not positive it needs a tune-up. Perhaps during this mental check-up is when you grab a blank sheet of paper to create your own, personalized Meditation on Words that is meaningful to you and your situation. A mental check-up may also help you understand which of the other practices you should commit to in order to release your negative thinking. (For me, it was realizing the need to forgive.)

I'm going to say this next part again: After you've created a Meditation on Words you need to *post it.* This is critical. It's the habitual part of the process after giving your brain a new synapse to fire by taking time to create the message in the first place. This repeated commitment is what designates this as a workout. If you don't take this step of posting your message for yourself, the old set of synapses firing off in their usual, negative fashion will take over, as they are a habit deeply engrained and strong. Be sure to place the messages you need your mind to see somewhere that it will see it every day, multiple times per day, including first thing in the morning (to jump start your new way of thinking) and last thing at night (to solidify your mindset before you succumb to sleep).

The first and foremost effect of trying a Meditation on Words is that you will immediately change the current negative context you are working within, because you have decided to do something *different*, no matter how small a change it may seem.

The second and ongoing effect of doing this is the habitual reminder of the positive to replace the habit of the negative. It's a constant interruption to your brain's bad habits with a message that is good.

As you feel this change in your mind, it will be as encouraging as if you were working out at the gym and seeing a change in your body: You'll want to do more of the positive. It gets more difficult to do unhealthy things for your self when you are habitually taking steps to try to take care of your self. As a relatable example for our bodies: It is harder for me to say "yes" to indulging in a sweet treat when I just worked hard for a month at the gym and was rewarded with dropping some pounds and feeling a looser fit to my jeans. Similarly, but from the mental perspective: I found it was harder for me to go negative in my mind, because I could now recognize it interrupting the happy place that I had finally gotten back to after so much dedicated work. Just like being healthy and fit was a result of the physical choices I would make each day, being happy and positive was a result of the mental choices I would make each day. It was *this* understanding that was the biggest lesson I learned along the way: My state of mind, both conscious and unconscious, was absolutely my choice, each and every moment, of each and every day. Once you learn and practice this habit, it's almost impossible to go back the other way. Happiness is your choice. A Meditation on Words is the workout you can do to help get yourself there.

I must admit this, to honor the fact that it's not just about thinking positively: There will have to be a coinciding process to unravel *why* you once decided to not live happily. This part certainly takes some time, so be patient with your self. For my personal situation I would say the practices toward positive thinking were my major focus for six months or more (until they became second nature once again, although I still tend to my brain every single day). Somewhere during that span of time there were many layers to work through of why and how I had become so overwhelmed and unhappy. I had to start by facing these things of the past, so that I could try to understand them from my renewed perspective, let go of my reasons to support these old ways of thinking and, in some cases, forgive ... so I could ultimately let these negative habits go. The collection of personal events leading to my collision was probably in the making for at least five years. I had created a lot of negative layers during that time; each one the building block for the next one layered on top. I recall visiting with Michele to share what I was discovering during this "uncovering" part of the process. She described the mental journey I was going through as similar to peeling back the thorny leaves of an artichoke, to get to the heart. It was an appropriate analogy.

The peeling back of my personal, thorny leaves started small and on the surface, with my statement of recognition and that preliminary visit to my doctor. This was followed by the immediate start of supplements and serotonin boosters (all over-the-counter), a trip home to seek the counsel and grounding comfort of my family, a meeting with my boss to communicate my troubles and re-set my boundaries (which had been entirely obliterated), a temporary but important adjustment to my work schedule to give me time to take care of myself (a later start each morning, out early each Friday), the practice of writing down lists of the plan and next steps (to get the thoughts disentangled from my confused mind), reading those written lists *often* to reinforce things for myself, going on many Thankful Walks, incorporating imagery exercises to help me stop my negative thoughts once they tried to start (I envisioned myself in boxing gloves and figuratively "punching out" the negative thoughts to stop them in their tracks), the regular practice of Meditation on Words, the practice of meditation by the light of a candle each morning, the practice of forgiveness three times a day for twenty-one days straight, and the reignited habit of going to church. Starting small enabled me to get stronger mentally, and prepared me to dig deeper into dealing with the reasons I had crashed to my low point.

As my mental habits started turning around it became a natural next step to bring into focus my physical habits: eating better, exercising regularly, stretching, not drinking as much, reaching out to my friends again, and making healthier, happier choices in general.

Soon thereafter other layers (which required more energy, which I was gaining more of each day) started to get addressed: I noticed that our home had fallen to the wayside, so I started not only taking better care of it, but creating a happy, peaceful surrounding for us to live in. I started taking better care in how I looked: dressing better, asking for a new hair style at the salon, getting back on track with the dentist and my oral health. I planted a garden and started planning fun events to look forward to.

Accomplishing the mental work to fix what was holding me down gave me renewed physical energy to jump onto this upward spiral and start to ride it once again. As each negative layer was taken away, and each new positive layer was brought in, I experienced the law of One-Thing-Leads-To-Another. I recognized that the majority of limits I faced were of my own making. The more I let go of those perceived limits, the greater my potential could be.

I was now on the exact opposite end of the spectrum from my crash to the bottom. The great testimony to that possibility of unlimited potential is the idea to write this book, to help anyone who might also be on the universal collision course with self. I have always desired to write a book and in this case I didn't have to try to write all this down; I simply couldn't avoid doing it.

My state of mind had turned around from dreading the start of each morning to wondering in each day what more could I do, and I am still in that state of mind to this day. Peeling back those thorny layers is the only way to get to the heart in earnest, be it the heart of the matter or just your happy heart as it's meant to be. Once you're there the rest comes naturally, and *the choice to be happy is yours for the making.*

CHAPTER FIVE

Images to Get You Started

(Don't just draw them – live them!)

No Negativity

Focus on the Positive

Simplify

Bring Balance Back into Your Life

Ask yourself first
before you try
to do
every little thing:

Is this
absolutely
necessary?

Less Work, More Fun

Less Indoors, More Outdoors

Take

Deep

Breaths

Stretch Your Body

Make Healthier Choices

Be aware of your thoughts;
keep your mind's
self-talk positive

Stop excessive worrying;
it is a waste
of your energy

There's a 50/50 chance
future circumstances
could turn
good or bad.
Choose to believe
the positive 50%

Expect the Best and plan for the Best!
(But know that stuff happens)

Focus on the things you are thankful for

Get back into the flow of your life

If you're holding
onto something
too tight,
practice
forgiveness

CHAPTER SIX

Why Stop There?

About six months into my process and following my initial visit home, my parents came to see me. This trip was originally planned as a touch-base to monitor how I was doing, as things were pretty dire at the time of my prior trip home to see them. My parents and Michele were all together in the same room with me one day, and openly talking about how far I'd come. I shared with them in detail the processes I practiced and heard often from them during this discussion the question of "Why stop there?" In other words, just because I had gotten myself out of my hole did not seem like enough of a reason to cease certain practices I had employed.

I clarified that I had not stopped all of them, and as an example explained that the twenty-one days of forgiveness was an excellent medicine for my condition. But after that particular practice and receiving the benefit from it, I didn't want to continue to bring attention to that aspect of my life any longer. The point was to be able to release and let it go. But I still was practicing healthy habits such as meditation each morning, reading *The Daily Word*, and creating new Meditations on Words to post to command central (while keeping the former posts still visible). In truth, those images on command central eventually started to get covered up by photos of family, friends, and fun events. But that had also been the point in the first place: I changed my perspective and day-to-day living from the negative to the positive, not only in my mind but in my life experience as well.

But the question "Why stop there?" reminded me of other images to use, to go beyond the basics of fixing my mindset, and take it to the next level of being the best I could be. The images to follow here are a very small and varied sampling of what that means.

These phrases and sayings have been offered to me by family and friends during the time it took me to write this book. They were shared by each of them while they worked through their own experiences—not at the basic level of trying to re-establish a positive mindset, but at the next level of using lifestyle habits to help navigate through whatever difficulties life may inevitably bring. To put it in context for you, the meaning of each phrase, as I understand it, is on the back of each page. These phrases strike me as each person's experience that can be universally helpful to all, and seemed like a perfect answer to the question "Why stop there?" They present another great opportunity to create your own personalized Meditation on Words, or utilize other methods of awareness, to help you be the best you imagine yourself to be.

CHAPTER SIX IMAGES:

Take It to the Next Level

Clean Up As You Go

Clean Up As You Go is the mantra of my dear friend Michele.
This phrase is the guiding light of her day-to-day life.
It is meant to include everything big and small in any given day,
from cleaning up your dishes as you use them,
to clarifying a communication that came out wrong,
to repairing any unintended damage in the relationships you share.
There is no sweeping of things under a rug
to tend to (or suffer from!) later
once you clean up as you go.

To Change Your Habits is to Change Your Mind

This was from a discussion between my dad and me, during his recovery phase after multiple surgeries. Now that he was out of the woods medically, it was time to fine tune his progress. After months of limited activity and a focus on the purely medical issues, he needed to start changing his basic eating and exercise habits back to a healthy and regular routine.

He had an extreme mental block toward changing his habits, but we talked and I reminded him of how focused he can be once he sets his mind to something. I sent him this Meditation on Words to post on his command central and remind him of that talk. I include it here as a reminder for anyone who needs to make the choice to change a habit that might be holding her or him back.

Throw open windows to the options of your Life

This is a Meditation on Words that was inspired by my doctor's advice to make important life decisions "from a position of strength and clarity." As I used her advice to work toward strength and clarity it made me realize two things: how constraining the current environment was that I was working within, and that it was up to me to break out of those constraints in order to live the life I imagined.

Communication

Is

Critical

This is a phrase adapted from friends working through various stages of their relationships, including long-time married couples, newlyweds, and singles who are dating. These folks share the commonality of being diligent to set aside time in their relationships for counseling, either for themselves individually, between themselves as a couple, or together with a third-party perspective. This is not necessarily because their relationship is in trouble, but because communication is complicated. Sometimes the simplest form of communication by one is loaded with a historical experience unknown to the other. These folks have learned if you are not clear and honest with your words, at all times, history can make the present moment cloudy. They practice their communication skills all the time, as a regular habit, and their relationships are the better for it.

Remember the Two-Hour Rule

This phrase came to me from a friend that had endured difficult times of unimaginable proportions, in losing her spouse to suicide. She had some dark days following that tragedy and found that she was shutting herself off completely from friends and loved ones, who were reaching out to her. She realized she had to stop automatically declining their invitations, because at some point they would stop asking. Losing her circle of support was as bad as accepting an invitation she might not be able to endure. So, she gave herself the "two-hour rule." This gave her the flexibility to say "yes" to friends reaching out to her, while allowing herself some latitude (and friends some forewarning) that if she was not up for it two hours prior to the event, she would be able to decline. This allowed her to manage her re-entry into the hustle and bustle of daily living, which seems to rarely give us a "time-out." It seems a useful rule that doesn't only need to be applied in times of extreme duress, but also while you are coming out of your own collision with self, or at any time that you are trying to create space for more flexibility and breathing room in the way you live.

Protect Your Personal Boundaries

This is adapted from a client who reminded me, "If you don't take care of yourself, who will?" This was in the context of sharing with each other how life can sometimes put you in "crisis mode," and that we are so connected these days, and so information-overloaded through technology, that the opportunity to be put in that position is greater than ever before. All of us may not have made the personal adjustments necessary to navigate efficiently through this age of the onslaught of technology, information, and being constantly connected. If you haven't done it yet, now is the time to define your personal boundaries and be your own ambassador for them. This will allow yourself the space to live the life you imagined.

More Romance

From my husband, as mentioned earlier in the book. A great reminder to make sure the business of life does not make your life feel like *all* business, especially for married couples. "Romance" can mean many different things—so decide what that might be for you or the two of you and bring it back into your life's picture!

CHAPTER SEVEN

The Quick List

Following is a list of the step-by-step actions I took, in the general order in which I took them, to help myself walk away from my collision feeling better than I ever had before. Some of these activities I still incorporate to this day and always will. They helped me become conscious of and thereby manage my state of mind. My improved state of mind led to much better decisions. Better decisions led to a happier day-to-day. A happier day-to-day has produced a happier life and I've found that a happier life is blessed with unlimited potential to live the life you've imagined!

Remember that these are the actions that worked for me and are meant to be a *guide for you to personalize* in ways that work for you. They are also meant to serve as a reminder to be patient, and that it will take time, determination, repetition, and multiple steps to get your self back on track.

Self-Acknowledgement ("I'm not okay")

Professional Help (Appointment with my doctor to address physical needs)

Seek Comforting Counsel (Visit home to be with my family and gather some strength)

Quiet Your Mind:

- Get It Out of Your Head (Write Lists: what the plan is, what the next steps of the plan are, how far you've come)

- Morning Meditation (I used the book *Handful of Quiet: Happiness in Four Pebbles* by Thich Nhat Hanh to help me get started)
- Deep-Breathing Practices
- Go For A Thankful Walk on a regular basis

Say a prayer every morning to set your mind before you start your day:

- Start with gratitude for your new awareness and for what is good in your life
- Ask for help with whatever is your need
- Focus on gaining and maintaining your peace from within
- Read *The Daily Word*

A Workout For Your Brain: Meditation on Words (create them and *post* them)

Simplify:

- Review Your Habits and use the "Is This Absolutely Necessary?" test
- This will help you pare down the "to do" list
- Try saying "no" or "Let me think about that" before you say "yes," to re-establish your personal boundaries
- Ensure more time for yourself—stop working so hard if it's at the expense of balance, health, and fun
- Disengage a little in order to re-engage consciously, with new habits
- Commit to a timeline of these simplifying practices (e.g., thirty days)
- Then review again and practice some more to adjust as necessary

Make no critical decisions until you are at a point of strength and clarity (e.g., quitting your job, leaving your marriage)

Practice Forgiveness, More of a Workout For Your Brain
(Three times per day for twenty-one days straight)

Attend Church
(Or some other gathering to soothe your soul and be surrounded by people in a peaceful state of mind)

Make Healthier Choices:

- Work out at whatever level suits you – as a statement that you are committed to doing good for yourself.
- Eat healthier—get conscious about what you are putting in your body.
- Review bad habits and commit to giving them a rest (drinking too much alcohol, too much caffeine, too many soft drinks, etc).
- As you eliminate bad habits, fill that space with good ones.

Build From There: Once you get on the positive updraft, the cycle of possibilities may surprise you!

CHAPTER EIGHT

The Ultimate Practice, "Second Best"

It seems that I should share this last chapter of the book for the benefit of the reader, even though this part of the story happened *before* my ultimate crash. I share it here hoping that other people, once they achieve the practice of how to tap into their mind and connect with their thoughts, can take that awareness to powerful levels of helping themselves. As an example of what I mean, my personal story goes like this.

For the majority of my adult life—well into my mid-thirties—I had this underlying self-image of being "second best." This perception comes from being born second in a family with a firstborn son who was "the golden child" (firstborn child, first grandson in the family on both sides, did everything by the book, etc.). But this perception also comes from my own childhood mind not being able to appropriately process certain key events at an early age, combined with taking too long in life to get back to that childhood perspective to review and understand it with an adult mind.

This "second best" perception permeated all the big choices I was making as I muddled my way through early adulthood. Where it became particularly visible—as pointed out by a very dear friend of mine—was in my selection of men (current husband not included). This friend, very kindly, did not see me as "second best" and was always stunned after hearing me talk highly about the latest love in my life, and consistently finding him to be not be anywhere near worthy of the bright light I had painted him in. In short, my friend always felt that I could do better and was consistently surprised that I could not see that for myself.

Other areas of my adult life that required major decision-making (e.g., employment and similar ways to advance myself) were also affected by this deeply engrained perception of being second best. It did not naturally occur to me to try to "rise to the top" in work situations; it only occurred to me to assist the person who would rise to the top.

Sometimes the examples of "second best" in my life were more subtle, and it took me time to realize that this was the force at play as I had painted myself into one of life's corners. But the problem reared its head often enough that I knew it was something I needed to address, by getting to the bottom of its source once and for all.

It was my friend Michele, not surprisingly, who pointed this out to me one day when I was struggling with one of the difficulties in my adult life. She recognized the "second best" force at play and called me out on it. I left my visit with Michele that day truly stunned, because she was right, and befuddled, because I thought I had dealt this nagging perception a final blow long ago by simply acknowledging it. As it turned out, acknowledging it wasn't enough ... I needed to *deal* with it.

As luck would have it, this visit with Michele happened on a Friday evening and I was about to have the entire weekend to myself with no particular plans. I drove home that night absolutely focused on this "second best" problem and determined to stay focused on it until I came to some sort of resolution. I was like a pit bull on a tire and frustrated as hell.

I spent that entire weekend at home taking care of mindless tasks so that I could keep my brain focused on *why* I continued to struggle with this "second best" conundrum. I found myself going from this most recent incident back to early years, highlighting particular moments that were the building blocks of this nagging perception. I remembered such things as returning home to visit the family (I live 2,500 miles away) and feeling "side-stepped" by my brother's entrance into our childhood home, even though he lives within an hour of the family. I remembered sitting down at the family dinner table on one of these visits home, feeling snubbed because my mother had forgotten to put out a place setting for me. I remembered what seemed like "unbalanced" treatments and/or punishments between my brother and me during our school years of testing the boundaries with our parents. On and on it went until I remembered the absolute foundational memory upon which I piled all of these building blocks of my "second best" perception.

I would estimate that I was about ten years old when this happened. My brother and I, as was our routine, had just spent two weeks of the summer with our grandparents at the Jersey Shore. While we were away our parents embarked upon the incredibly ambitious project of completely re-doing our childhood rooms: new wallpaper, new carpet, new bedspreads—the works. This was meant to be a surprise to my brother and me, only to be discovered upon walking into our bedrooms when we got home. My ten-year-old mind's memory recorded the scene like this: I was sitting alone on the new carpet of my bedroom, while both of my parents were in the adjacent bedroom with my brother enjoying his reaction to all of their hard work. Feeling dejected I cried out, "You love him more than me!" only to be answered with "Janice, be quiet." You can understand how this memory would be significant to someone with only ten years of experience to process it in any kind of useful manner.

While I was thinking on this memory during this particular weekend spent in my home, an image suddenly flashed to my mind—and I recognized it to be significant right away. It was not unlike seeing an image behind your eyelids when you close them after looking out the window for a spell ... shadows of light and dark, but a definite image ... like the old-time negatives of photography.

I quickly went upstairs and found that same sketch pad from college I mentioned in the beginning of this book, and started drawing the image I saw in my mind. I could not believe what it was when I was done: the image of both of my parents, in my newly updated childhood room, sitting together with terrific smiles on their face, waiting for me to see their loving work for the very first time.

What I realized about this image is this is how it *actually* happened, but my mind had decided to truncate the memory and remember it wrong. I remembered it clearly now: both of my parents in my room with me *first*, knowing how important a young girl's room is to her. It was my brother who was alone in his room waiting for them to visit, after they *first* shared the moment with me. When they left me to go visit him is when I sat on the floor and felt dejected, because I still (selfishly) wanted their company, and that was the only emotion my ten-year-old mind decided to remember in a solitary way. But in actuality, they were with me *first*.

This was a profound moment for me in my adult life, sitting alone in my house and staring at the sketch. I had *created* that "second best" perception and built upon it for *decades*, all because I remembered that early scene of my life incorrectly. I was stunned and, to be honest, embarrassed as well as shocked at the power of my created reality.

I knew that I needed to see this sketch *every single day* in order to un-do the two decades of original memory habit in my brain, so I hung the picture on my closet door where I would see it every morning while getting dressed to leave the house. It still hangs there today, but I know its work is done. That "second best" perception is history, my life choices are reflective of that, and my memory has been set straight forever.

It was this experience that originally started my education about my relationship to my brain, the impact of meditating on words and (in this case) images, and how we have the power to work with our minds—even decades after an initial event. I had no idea of just how far I would need to take this education, after experiencing my collision with self. But I am thankful I had this awareness beforehand so that I could acknowledge that I "wasn't okay" before things got out of my reach. I should mention here that I have spent many times before trying to get to the root of that damaging, underlying perception. As with all things mentioned in this book, the process takes time. But I also wanted you to know that it works, and that we have incredible power to tap into ourselves in order to not only capitalize upon the things that are working well for us, but also to do away with the things that are taking away from us. The choice to do so is yours for the making, and that's the most powerful part.

CHAPTER NINE

Conclusion – Back to Reality

The writing of this book took more than a year. I've had the opportunity to monitor and examine my new way of engaging with "the real world" since the uprising from my initial collision. Here's what my experience has taught me thus far.

On occasion, those old, negative synapses will start to fire off again to affect my day and how I operate in the world. The good news is that I now recognize this almost immediately so that I can arrest that old habit as it starts and take action to get my positive mindset back to the forefront. Often that means I need to take a couple of minutes to do a deep-breathing practice, a practice of forgiveness (if it applies), or a silent prayer.

The world remains fast-paced and multi-faceted in the ways we communicate, and our personal boundaries are constantly threatened. In fact, there is no regard for them at all in this technological age; it is a boundary each of us bears the responsibility to set for our own selves. I am much more aware of this now than I was prior to the crash, and that experience has taught me to be vigilant. Remember that a combination of overages will have its consequences.

In addition to moderating my intake of various media sources, I am much more diligent now with my "is this absolutely necessary?" test in my other day-to-day decisions. I learned there was a lot I felt responsible for that could be eliminated. Not everything on my "to do" list was truly necessary; they were often just habits that needed re-examination. I am aware of and thoughtful with every choice I make within the course of each day.

I've learned that we need to have a "mental garage sale" every now and then, in order to keep a crash at bay. Just like cleaning out the physical junk in my garage gives me more space to work with, cleaning out the mental junk in my brain seems to have had the same effect: I feel like I have much more room in there now. On my way to the collision with my self I felt like I was constantly running into hurdles and stumbling along in the day-to-day activities of my world. I was quite frankly so muddled and clouded that there was really no other option. Now I am engaged in what is happening around me every day and I feel I am flowing, instead of constantly hitting walls. I am picking up on messages in conversation with others that are important to my long-term goals. I am running into new people who have a new perspective to offer that helps guide my way. Before, I could barely keep up my end of a social conversation, if I chose to engage with others at all. Now I feel like I am living my life with a specific intent. It is the complete and exact opposite of feeling as if I am floating away like a helium balloon.

But the last part that I now understand is the greatest testimonial possible for making sure this book is available to all: Our society is not well-trained to keep a sympathetic eye open to mental distress. This statement held true for the management team of my division, who were wonderful to give me a minor adjustment in my schedule when I crashed, but had no precedent to guide them in maintaining a consistent understanding during my recovery. I would say they were simply doing the best they could with limited experience in this regard. As an example, a couple of months into my adjusted schedule they came back to me to say that others in my place of work were feeling that they were now owed an adjustment to their schedules as well, indicating that it was time for me to get it together. Had we all had a better precedent to work from it would have been easier for others to understand that, while not a tangible recovery process (such as an appointment for a physical therapy session each morning), it was still a process that took time, that I could not get it together based on a known timeline, and that communication (to the extent allowable) with the team would likely have gone a long way toward a better understanding for all. This experience has made apparent to me that mental struggles are often overlooked and/or misunderstood, and people in need of help are often left to their own devices.

These mental attacks on our bodies can be just as serious as, if not more so than, physical ones. Both can be equally devastating, if not as equally obvious. I happen to live in an area of the nation that has one of the highest rates of suicide, and know more than my fair share of successful suicide attempts. Though I never got to the point of actually planning harm to myself, I did have moments of passive acts of checking out (which I did discuss with my doctor): "If that bus hit me, it would be okay" and other thoughts similar to that. I absolutely can see how someone would get to the point of deciding to take their life in order to end the despairing perspective of "So, this is how the rest of my days are going to be?" I am aware of my good fortune to have already been enough in tune with myself to recognize "I'm not okay," before that downward spiral got out of my reach. I had enough of a glimpse of the truly dark side to help me understand how it can happen, and does happen, for so many people.

Which brings me back to Michele, the friend in my life who did have the experience, open mind, and loving heart to be worried for my well-being, long before I was. She let me know about her concern multiple times over many years. I'm forever grateful to her and will use her as a role model of how I will live my years going forward. If I see someone on a self-collision course (and I do recognize it now more than ever before) I'm stepping up. I'm going to say something, even if it doesn't go well. I'm going to keep tabs on that person and I'm not going to turn a blind eye. I'm going to ask them the questions that need to be asked, and I'm going to offer advice and help if I have them to give. If I don't, I will encourage them to get in front of someone who does.

It's a good challenge to take, and I lay it on the table for all of us to accept. Leaving someone that is in a pained state of mind to their own devices does not seem to be working well for our society at large. I would advocate for some sort of program in the schools to help teens understand the power of their state of mind, before they decide the only answer to their angst is to gun down their schoolmates. In my decades of adulthood thus far I've seen our society become more compassionate and accepting of things that were not openly talked about during my childhood years. *Mental health is the next subject for us to bring into focus.*

Because in all sincerity, it comes down to this: We never know what twists and turns Life may have in store for us, and which end of the mental health spectrum we may find ourselves on, the one where we need help or the one where we can offer it. So it seems best to be prepared for both by setting a precedent of sympathy for others, tending to our own state of mental health and awareness, and helping others to do the same.

Good luck to you, dear Reader … you can do this!

APPENDIX

This appendix contains some of the actual images I drew as part of my personal Meditation on Words. I wanted the reader to see that they are not of any kind of artistic quality or skill, to emphasize that artistic talent is not the point. The point is the practice of meditating on positive thoughts, and the repetition of the messages for your brain, to provide it the workout that it needs to get back to a state of positive mental health.

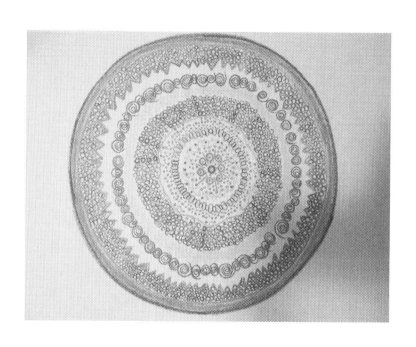

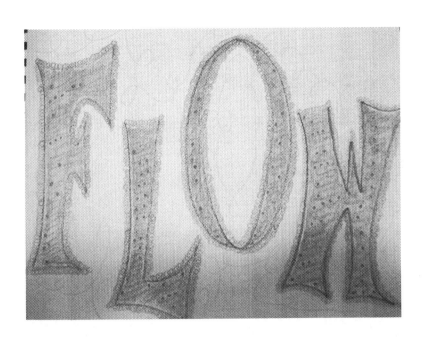

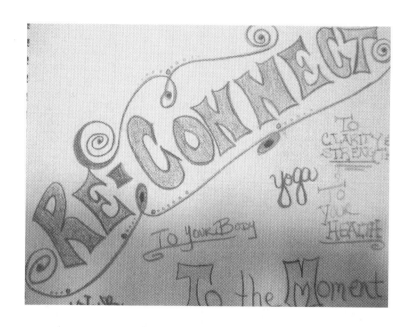

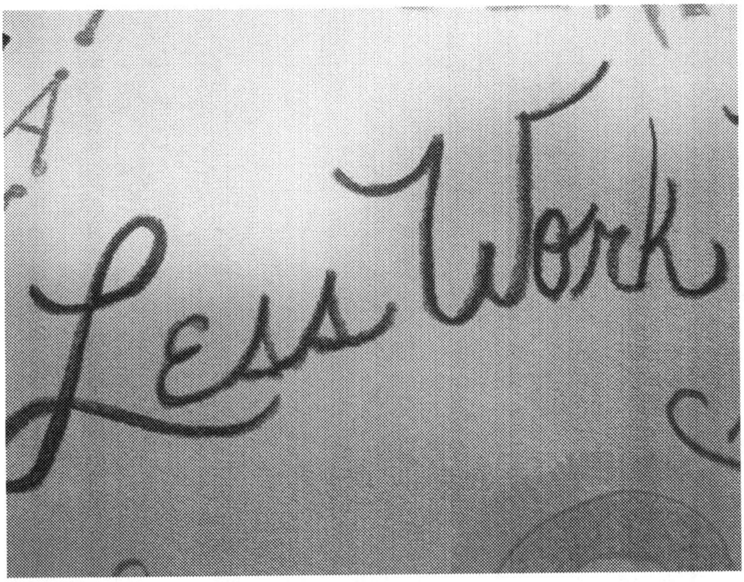
Less Work

More Fun!

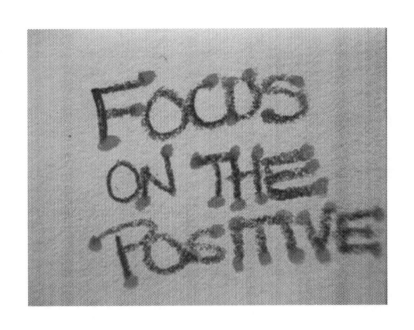

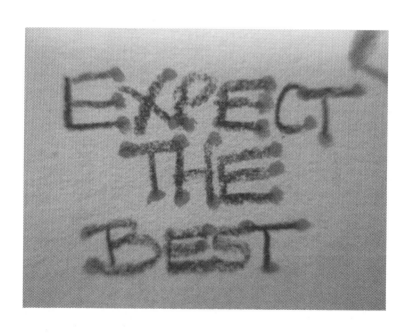

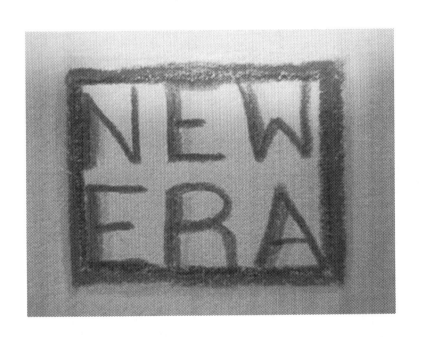

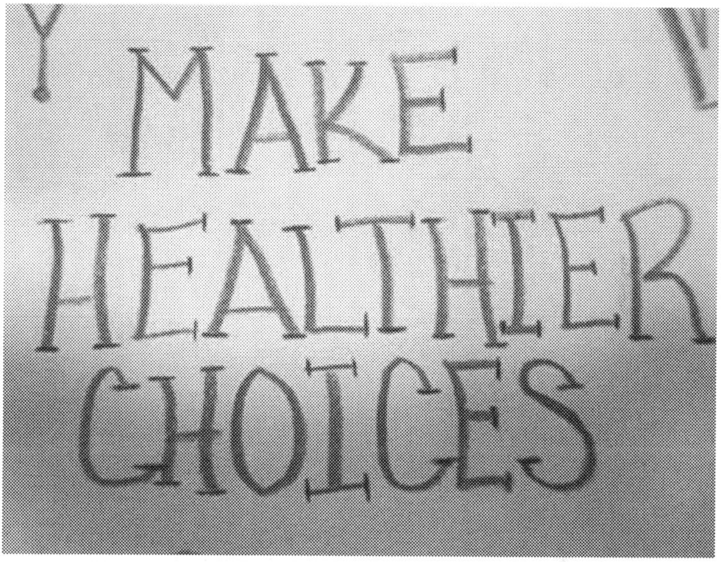
MAKE
HEALTHIER
CHOICES

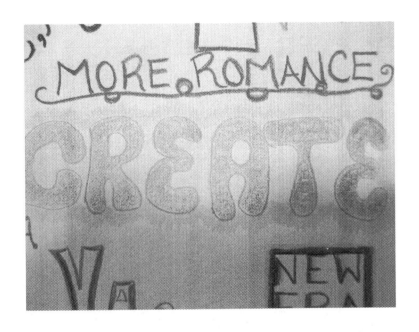

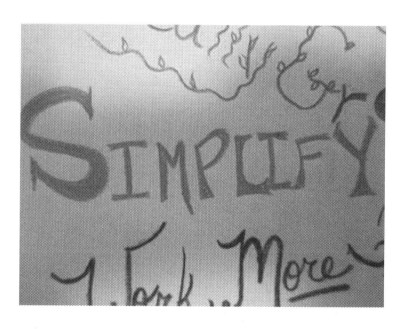

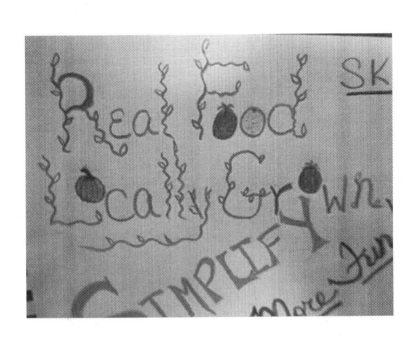

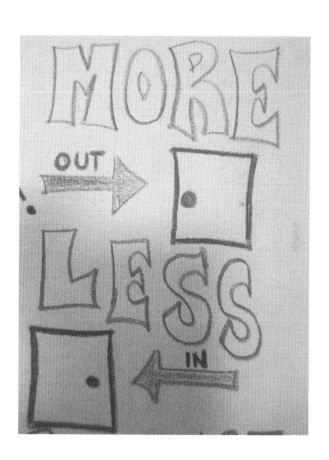

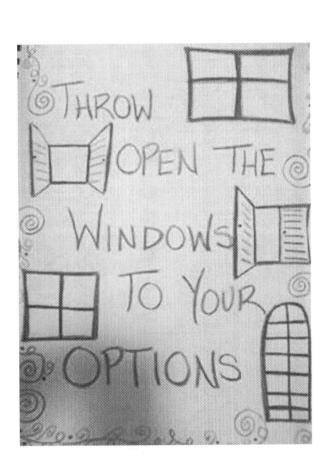

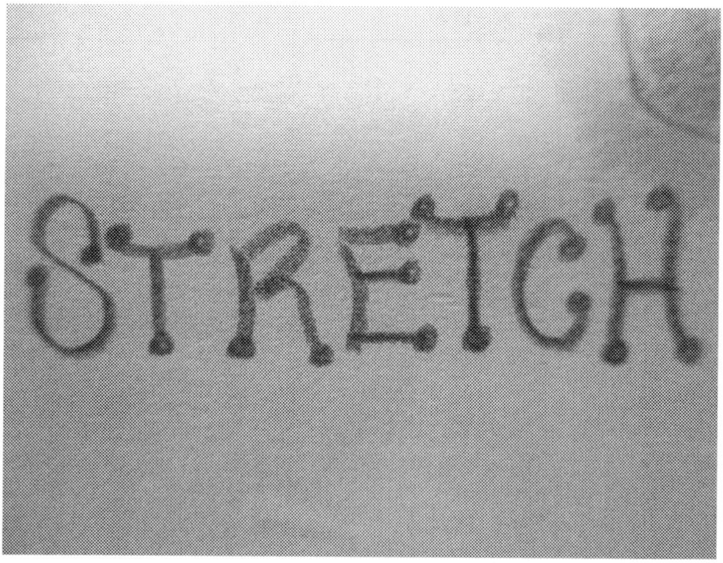
STRETCH

Official contact information for *The Daily Word*: Unity World Headquarters at Unity Village, 1901 NW Blue Parkway, Unity Village, MO 64065-0001, www.dailyword.com.

Books of Encouragement: *A Handful of Quiet: Happiness in Four Pebbles*, by Thich Nhat Hanh; *A Short Guide to a Happy Life*, by Anna Quindlen; *Who Moved My Cheese?* by Spencer Johnson, M.D.

ABOUT THE AUTHOR

Janice Daler was born and raised in New Jersey and now lives in Colorado with her husband. She graduated from Rutgers University with dual degrees in English and Communications, and she later earned her designation as a Certified Trust and Financial Advisor from a premier financial institute. This is her first book and was written solely with the intent to help others.